# I'M NOT WEIRDO
# I JUST HAVE ASPERGER

## Discovering the beauty of a different world

**José Ricardo Cantú Aguilar**

# INDEX

## Content


Introduction .................................................................................................... 3

Chapter 1: Background of Psychosocial Disability ..................................... 7

Chapter 2: Neurotypicals ........................................................................... 11

Chapter 3: Autism ...................................................................................... 17

Chapter 4: Asperger .................................................................................. 22

Chapter 5: Do We Really Choose Who We Are? ...................................... 30

Chapter 6: The Difference Between Tolerance and Inclusion ................. 35

Chapter 7: Life with Asperger's ............................................................... 43

Chapter 8: What to Do in an Autistic Crisis ............................................ 49

Chapter 9: Feeling Whole While Being Alone .......................................... 57

Chapter 10: Cure it? Treat it? Control it? NO...understand it. ............... 62

Chapter 11: Anecdotes ............................................................................. 71

Final Chapter: Thank you very much to all my readers! ....................... 113

Poems about Autism and Its Derivatives ............................................... 116

Final Acknowledgments ........................................................................... 121

Dear Mom,

I know you're worried about me. I know you've noticed that there are some things about me that are different from others. I try my best to adapt, but it's not always easy. You might think I'm antisocial because I don't want to go to parties, but that doesn't mean I don't want to have friends; I'm just scared of being around too many people. You might think I'm a coward for being a pacifist, but that doesn't mean I don't know how to defend myself; I just can't understand when someone speaks ill of me. You might think I'm selfish, but that doesn't mean I don't care about others; it's just hard for me to understand how to act in every situation. It's difficult for me to understand others or even comprehend what's happening around me. No matter how hard I try, I've never been able to fit into this society. But... you know what? I don't want to feel bad for being different anymore, and I don't want to remain depressed because of my social relationships. I have fought for a better future, and I am truly proud of everything I've achieved so far and what I know I will achieve in the future, despite being judged for who I am by my friends, classmates, teachers, or even my own family.

Despite everything, Mom, it makes me feel better knowing that even if you don't fully understand me, you're always there to support me. You explain things to me when I'm confused, and you allow me to express my feelings safely. It's possible that on more than one occasion, I've made you feel like you're not important to me, and that's why I want you to know that, in my own way, I love you unconditionally. I promise that everything I achieve will be thanks to you, even if I have to move mountains and seas to make the world understand that I'm not a weirdo; I just have Asperger's.

Have you ever felt different from others? Have you felt out of place among classmates, coworkers, or even your own family? Do you find it difficult to converse with other people? Do you struggle to understand jokes or double meanings? Have more than one person called you weird? Then we recommend reading this book, where we explain that being "weird" doesn't necessarily mean something bad; it can be the perfect opportunity to understand that you are just different from others because... you might have Asperger's

Asperger's is a unique condition that affects many people around the world. This condition is characterized by difficulties with social skills, language skills, and an intense interest in a specific subject. While many people with Asperger's are capable of leading fulfilling lives, many also struggle to cope with the diagnosis and its consequences

This book will address the topic of Asperger's from various angles. We will explore the symptoms often associated with the disorder, the challenges people with Asperger's face, and how they can receive support both at home and in the school environment. Additionally, we will discuss the available treatments to help individuals with Asperger's reach their full potential.

Throughout the book, we will cover the condition from all perspectives and emphasize the importance of understanding and respecting people with Asperger's. We will encourage everyone to recognize their strengths and support them in their attempts to find their own path. Our main goal is to remind those involved that they are not alone, and despite all the sacrifices, there will always be hope for a better future.

# Chapter 1: Background of Psychosocial Disability

Psychosocial disability has become one of the socially accepted concepts of today; however, its background dates back to ancient times. Before the term autism was coined, it was difficult to diagnose and identify certain characteristics and difficulties related to behavior and development. Initially, children with autism spectrum disorders (ASD) were thought to be "abnormal" in some way and were considered incapable of reaching their potential to develop properly. Many children with ASD were rejected due to society's ignorance, rejection, and stigma. For example, in the late 19th and early 20th centuries, some parents were terrified to see their children with ASD. These children were perceived as mentally retarded, so it was common for parents to leave them in institutions where they were cared for, isolated from the rest of society.

These children were considered abnormal, which led many parents to feel ashamed of their children. This social conception also led children with ASD to receive extreme treatments such as shock therapies and sometimes forced physical treatments, all with the aim of curing them or improving their behavior. Fortunately, social conception has changed a lot since then, and it is now understood that autism is not a disease but a developmental condition.

Children with ASD now receive better treatments, such as behavioral therapy, occupational therapy, speech therapy, and music therapy. These treatments help children reach their full potential, bringing them closer to the rest of society.

In the 18th century, mental disorders began to be studied in more detail thanks to the famous "Enlightenment," an intellectual movement that advocated for rationality and the use of reason as the primary method for achieving progress. During this period, the concept of mental disability began to emerge, and numerous scientific studies on the subject were conducted.

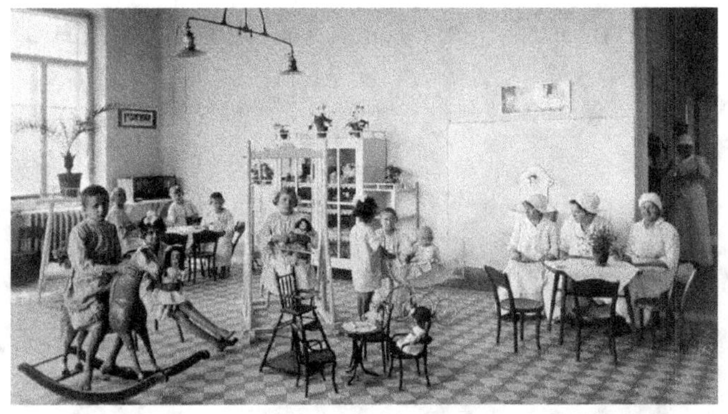

Children with Autism Admitted to a Psychiatric Hospital in the 20th Century

In the 19th century, mental disorders were recognized as an illness and later as a disability. Government laws were adapted to consider the rights of people with intellectual, mental, and psychosocial disabilities, and the first efforts were made to provide special services for them.

Subsequently, in the 20th century, advances in the field of psychiatry allowed for the diagnosis and treatment of psychosocial disorders. Cognitive-behavioral therapies enabled the treatment of psychosocial disabilities, and prevention programs were established to prevent the emergence of new disabilities.

Today, psychosocial disability is recognized as a condition that can be treated with the help of modern medical advances and the efforts of mental health professionals to improve the quality of life for those

who suffer from it.

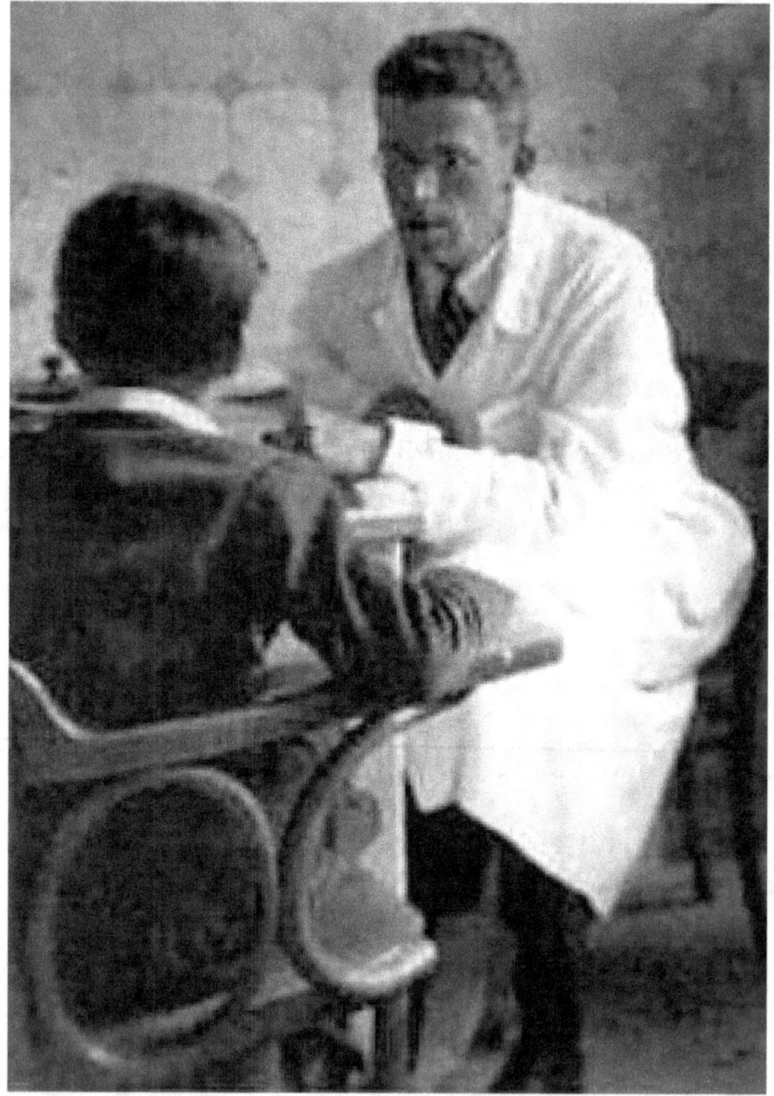

Hans Asperger conducting experiments on the detection and behavior of autism in
children.

# Chapter 2: Neurotypicals

*"Neurotypicals simply assume that they are the teachers, and we are the students when it comes to appropriate behavior."*

While it is not a commonly used term to the extent that it is not even considered an official word in the Royal Spanish Academy (RAE), it is widely used in the scientific community (especially among psychologists and psychiatrists). The truth is that it is very likely that you, as readers, are an example of the word "neurotypical." A neurotypical person is someone who does not have any syndrome or disorder that can affect their daily life, whether in physical, psychological, or social matters.

In recent years, there have been various debates about the term neurotypical. Firstly, some experts claim that it is practically impossible for more than 10% of the world's population to be declared 100% neurotypical today. As the global population has increased in recent decades and as new technologies have developed for (or against) human interaction (i.e., social media and the internet), humans have significantly developed various disorders such as anxiety, depression, attention deficit hyperactivity disorder (ADHD), stress, narcissistic personality disorder, or syndromes such as Paranoid Personality Disorder (PPD). Another debate that has gained traction in recent years discusses the possibility that more people with some disorder or syndrome have been born in the new millennium. In a way, it is correct to say that there are more people today who cannot be declared neurotypical, primarily due to the excessive use of social media and trends, as well as the drastic increase in the world's population, which now has over 8 billion inhabitants.

On the other hand, as technology has advanced, new scientific discoveries have been made about the functioning of the human brain. This has led to the development of new methods for identifying various neurological disorders in children and adults, whether in school, family, or even in the work environment. Therefore, it would be more accurate to say not simply that there are fewer neurotypicals than before but that it is easier to detect disorders compared to past decades. The biggest mistake a neurotypical person can make is to judge other personalities and label them as "weird" or "crazy" without considering whether their counterparts have been diagnosed with some type of disorder. Usually, people who are most often labeled as "weird" are those diagnosed with Autism Spectrum Disorder (ASD) and Attention Deficit Hyperactivity Disorder (ADHD).

One of the most interesting aspects of neurotypicals is the way society tends to idealize and value their characteristics and abilities. Neurotypical individuals are often the benchmark for measuring "normalcy," and others, particularly those with neurological differences, are expected to conform to these standards. This can lead to the marginalization and discrimination of those who do not fit this mold, highlighting the importance of understanding and promoting neurodiversity.

On the other hand, empathy and theory of mind—the ability to put oneself in others' shoes and understand their thoughts and emotions—are skills that are usually well-developed in neurotypicals. This facilitates the building of interpersonal relationships and collaboration in social and work environments. Most neurotypical individuals also have well-developed verbal language and communication, enabling them to express their thoughts and feelings effectively.

In terms of education and employment, neurotypicals often benefit from systems designed for their needs and preferences. Schools and workplaces are frequently structured according to typical communication skills and learning styles, which can create challenges for those who are neurodiverse. This raises the question of how to adapt and diversify educational and workplace environments to better accommodate all individuals, regardless of their neurotypicality.

The role of a neurotypical in society is fundamental, but it is essential to understand that diversity in neurological functioning is a natural characteristic of humanity. Valuing neurodiversity and promoting inclusive environments is a crucial step towards a more just and understanding society for everyone, regardless of their neurotypicality.

Additionally, it's important to recognize that neurotypicals also have their own unique challenges and experiences. Not every neurotypical individual fits perfectly into societal norms, and many face difficulties that require support and understanding. By fostering an inclusive mindset, we can create a world where everyone's experiences are validated and respected.

Promoting awareness and education about neurodiversity can lead to more supportive communities. Schools can implement programs that teach children about different neurological conditions, helping to build empathy and reduce bullying. Workplaces can provide training for employees to better understand and accommodate their neurodiverse colleagues, fostering a more inclusive and productive work environment.

Inclusion also extends to policy-making. Governments and institutions can develop policies that protect the rights of neurodiverse individuals and ensure they have access to necessary resources and accommodations. This holistic approach can contribute to a society that not only accepts but celebrates the full spectrum of human diversity.

Ultimately, understanding neurotypicality and neurodiversity is a step towards a more compassionate and equitable society. By valuing each person's unique contributions and providing the support they need, we can create an environment where everyone has the opportunity to thrive.

# Chapter 3: Autism

*"Autism is proof that love doesn't need words. Asperger's is an opportunity to explore the world in new and innovative ways."*

Have You Ever Put Yourself in the Shoes of an Autistic Person? Autism can be a challenge for those who have it, as well as for their families, friends, and caregivers. It is a complex disorder that affects a person's ability to communicate, interact with others, understand social behavior, and respond to their environment. Autism is not a disease, but rather a developmental condition present from birth.

First, it is important to understand the difference between autism and intellectual disability. Autism is a developmental disorder that affects social, communicative, and cognitive functioning. This means that individuals with autism may have difficulties establishing interpersonal connections and understanding language and gestures, in addition to having problems learning and processing information. Intellectual disability, on the other hand, refers to reduced intellectual capabilities and academic functioning, which may or may not be accompanied by behavioral problems.

Furthermore, autism manifests in different degrees and symptoms, meaning that each individual affected by this disorder will have a unique experience. This implies that managing autism symptoms must be personalized according to each person's specific needs. Some people with autism may easily demonstrate this condition, while others may have managed their symptoms so effectively that it is hard to believe they have the condition.

There are several therapies that can help individuals with autism and their families. These therapies focus on improving the individual's social, communicative, and intellectual skills. They include cognitive-behavioral therapy, acceptance and commitment therapy, play therapy, life skills training, speech therapy, among others. These therapies can help individuals with autism improve their ability to communicate and relate to others.

It is also important for family members, caregivers, and the general environment to be aware of the challenges faced by a person with autism and the problems they experience. This includes being attentive and understanding the behavior patterns and symptoms of autism, as well as offering support and understanding. Empathy and patience are key to fostering a supportive environment, which can help improve the quality of life for the person with autism.

Commonly, people who are not familiar with Asperger's or autism tend to show aggressive, disrespectful, or indifferent behavior towards patients. This is because the empathy of an average person is often limited to those who display similar behavior patterns to what they are accustomed to. Any variation or anomaly in behavior can create negative thoughts from the neurotypical person towards their counterpart. While the word "acceptance" might be easy to consider in theory, in practice, it is challenging to follow through. Therefore, being empathetic and patient is crucial for the development of individuals with autism.

Understanding autism also involves recognizing the strengths and unique abilities of individuals with the condition. Many people with autism have exceptional skills in specific areas such as mathematics, music, art, or memory. These strengths should be encouraged and developed, as they can provide a sense of accomplishment and purpose.

Public awareness and education about autism are also crucial. By spreading knowledge and understanding about the condition, society can become more inclusive and supportive. Schools, workplaces, and communities can implement programs and policies that accommodate the needs of individuals with autism, making it easier for them to integrate and participate fully in society.

Moreover, early diagnosis and intervention are essential. The earlier autism is identified, the sooner interventions can begin, which can significantly improve outcomes for individuals with autism. Parents and caregivers should be informed about the signs of autism and seek professional advice if they have concerns about their child's development.

In conclusion, while autism presents significant challenges, it also offers an opportunity to see the world from a different perspective. By fostering empathy, understanding, and support, society can create an environment where individuals with autism can thrive and reach their full potential.

# Chapter 4: Asperger

*"Imagine you are in a bustling foreign city at night, crowded with people, unable to understand the language being spoken, recognizing only a few words but not fully comprehending them, just like the situations happening around you. You feel the need to ask for help, but you can't. This experience can start to help you understand what a child, teenager, or adult with Asperger's feels on an ordinary day."*

In this chapter, we will explain in detail Autism Spectrum Disorder (ASD) and its different levels: Asperger's, Rett syndrome, atypical autism syndrome (ATA), and classic infantile autism. We will discuss the developmental factors that can contribute to the disorder and provide a clear definition of the symptoms associated with Asperger's. This will include a detailed discussion of the difficulties with social skills and language often found in Asperger's. Finally, we will examine the factors that differentiate Asperger's from classic autism.

Asperger Syndrome (AS) is a developmental disorder particularly related to language and social interaction, primarily affecting boys and adults. The term was coined by Dr. Hans Asperger in 1944, although the characteristics of Asperger's were described much earlier.

Deviating a bit from the topic and mentioning Hans Asperger, I would like to tell you a little about this figure: Friedrich Hans Asperger was an Austrian doctor recognized for his work in the field of autism. He was the first to theorize about Asperger syndrome in 1944, which is known as the first modern work on the topic. In fact, he was one of the first to use the term "Autism Spectrum Disorder (ASD)." Before Asperger, cases of autism were treated as separate and isolated syndromes, without understanding that they were part of a unique entity. This lack of understanding made it difficult to effectively identify and treat patients.

During the 1940s, Asperger was the most recognized scientist for the study and description of what is now known as Asperger's syndrome. He studied and cataloged, in great detail, the behaviors, attitudes, and abilities of patients with autism. He described how cases of autism differ among themselves and how this affected the level of social, cognitive, mental, sensory, and communicative skills of the patients.

Asperger's work greatly helped to provide a better understanding of the different types of autism and opened the door for better treatment. This allowed people with autism and their families to feel understood and professionals to find a better path to handle these situations.

Today, people with Asperger's syndrome especially benefit from Hans Asperger's work, as adaptation mechanisms have been developed that allow these individuals to improve their social skills, as well as facilitate the identification and treatment of their needs.

On the other hand, this Austrian pediatrician has also been a controversial figure in the history of medicine. Although his studies and observations have been fundamental in understanding autism and variations in neurological development, his legacy is tainted by his behavior and affiliations during World War II.

During this period, Asperger worked within a medical system deeply intertwined with Nazi ideology. His involvement in the Third Reich's eugenics program, which promoted the elimination of individuals deemed "undesirable" due to their disability or medical condition, has been a subject of intense scrutiny and condemnation. Historical documents and recent studies reveal that Asperger supported the Nazis' "racial hygiene" policies and collaborated in identifying children with disabilities for subsequent extermination in child euthanasia programs, such as the infamous Am Spiegelgrund, a clinic in Vienna where horrific practices were carried out.

Additionally, Asperger was known for his nationalist sentiments in favor of Germany and his alignment with the Third Reich's ideology. Although he has been credited with attempting to protect some children from Nazi persecution by labeling them as "valuable," his complicity with the regime and its genocidal policies cannot be overlooked.

This grim aspect of Hans Asperger's life has led to his being considered a "persona non grata" in many communities. The reevaluation of his legacy highlights the importance of examining not only a person's scientific contributions but also their ethics and the context in which they operated. Recognizing and confronting these dark aspects is essential to honor the victims and ensure that history does not repeat itself. Thus, while we continue to use the term "Asperger syndrome" for its clinical and descriptive value, it is crucial to remember and learn from the complexities and controversies of its origin.

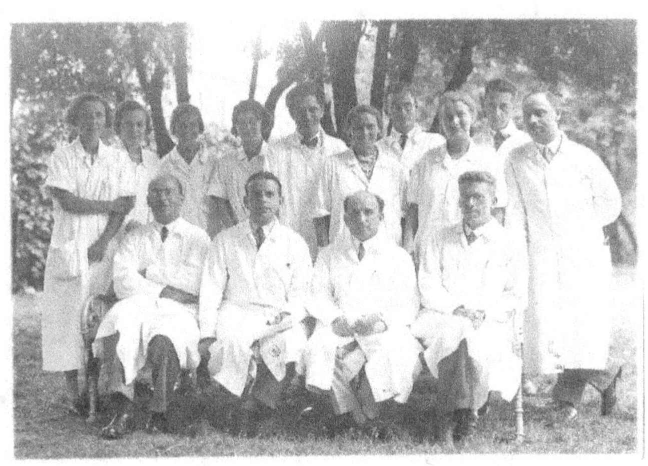

Hans Asperger and his team

Returning to the initial topic, Asperger described the syndrome as an "intermediate" form between psychopathy and autism. In subsequent years, further research demonstrated that Asperger's syndrome occurs when a person exhibits characteristics of autism but to a much lesser degree. The symptoms of Asperger's are variable, with some children displaying brilliant abilities in certain areas, while others face greater difficulties in maintaining contact with others.

Children with Asperger's syndrome generally have a family history of neurological issues, such as epilepsy, Gilles de la Tourette syndrome, dyslexia, paranoid personality disorder, or even Tourette's syndrome.

People with Asperger's syndrome have difficulties interacting with others and may even feel intimidated or frustrated in social environments, particularly when encountering new people. These individuals often struggle to understand social cues, such as body language, humor, metaphors, and cultural differences. These difficulties can significantly impact the formation of friendships and relationships with peers.

Moreover, individuals with this condition also have trouble understanding and using spoken language. This can pose challenges in conversations, classes, and social situations. Verbal language, comprehension, and the use of nonverbal language are specific areas where many children with autism face problems. However, in the case of Asperger's, most patients exhibit highly formal and grammatically correct speech even from a young age, making it easier to identify them among other children.

Despite these limitations, Asperger's syndrome is often considered more of a difference or condition than a disability. Many children and adults with this syndrome have exceptional skills and talents in areas such as music, mathematics, art, and computer science. There are even numerous cases of patients with excellent photographic and/or auditory memory who tend to identify details with greater ease than a neurotypical individual. These talents are often used as a way to compensate for some of their social difficulties.

An important point that people often overlook is that, unlike other mental disorders like Down syndrome, it is not really known how or why Asperger's syndrome develops in fetuses. It is crucial to remember that a person is born, lives, and dies with Asperger's. Since it is not known how it develops, it is also unknown how to treat it effectively. In simple terms, Asperger's has no cure or treatment because it is not a disease but something one is born with, just like being neurotypical. Therefore, Asperger's should be understood and accepted.

# Chapter 5: Do We Really Choose Who We Are?

*Who among us is "normal" enough to decide what is truly considered "normal" or not? Don't worry about trying to be what is called "normal" because some people talk about it only because they don't know the feeling of being unique and not just another "copy."*

It is an axiom that every human being is unique, that each of us has different goals, aspirations, and dreams, as well as opinions, feelings, and/or knowledge that vary depending on the topic. This individuality is shaped by various factors such as the culture instilled by our parents, the things we learned during our formative years, the people we met and formed bonds with, whether in love or friendship, whose teachings may or may not have influenced our development, goals, or worldview, the country we live in, the era we were born in, the events we may have experienced in our respective lives, and even the things we may have seen and/or heard at some point in our lives that might have made us reflect on one or more specific topics, causing a series of events in the future.

Despite being proud of our individuality, the truth is that humans follow a series of physical and mental patterns, whether with our own species or even with other species, that make us question at certain points in our lives: "Are we really unique?" or "Do we really have free will?"

While we have physical differences (such as our fingerprints) and mental differences (such as our own existential rationality) that could in some way give us that individuality and special characteristic that makes us unique, the truth is that on a planet where more than eight billion humans live and interact, it would be difficult, if not impossible, for there not to be at least one person who is exactly the same as us both physically and mentally.

Far from seeming like fiction, the truth is that at least in the physical aspect, it is proven that we can have almost exact replicas of ourselves living in other parts of our planet, country, or even our own city, whether of the same gender or the opposite gender.

An example of this is the famous Canadian photographer François Brunelle, who has dedicated the last two decades to searching for and photographing people who share identical physical traits but are not related by family; that is, they were born to different families yet still share the same physical identity.

Over the past two decades, the artist not only demonstrated that identical people can exist who were born in different parts of the world, but also, when interviewing and conducting photography sessions with them, he was surprised to learn that in most cases, his models displayed very similar behaviors and opinions, and in a few cases, completely identical ones. For the photographer, it was incredible to see two different people sharing the same tastes, the same opinions, the same expressions, and even similar voices, despite having had different lives and families.

That said, and returning to the initial topic, while as human beings we might say that we have certain characteristics that could make us truly unique, the truth is that out there, there are potential candidates who could be up to 99% identical to us both physically and mentally.

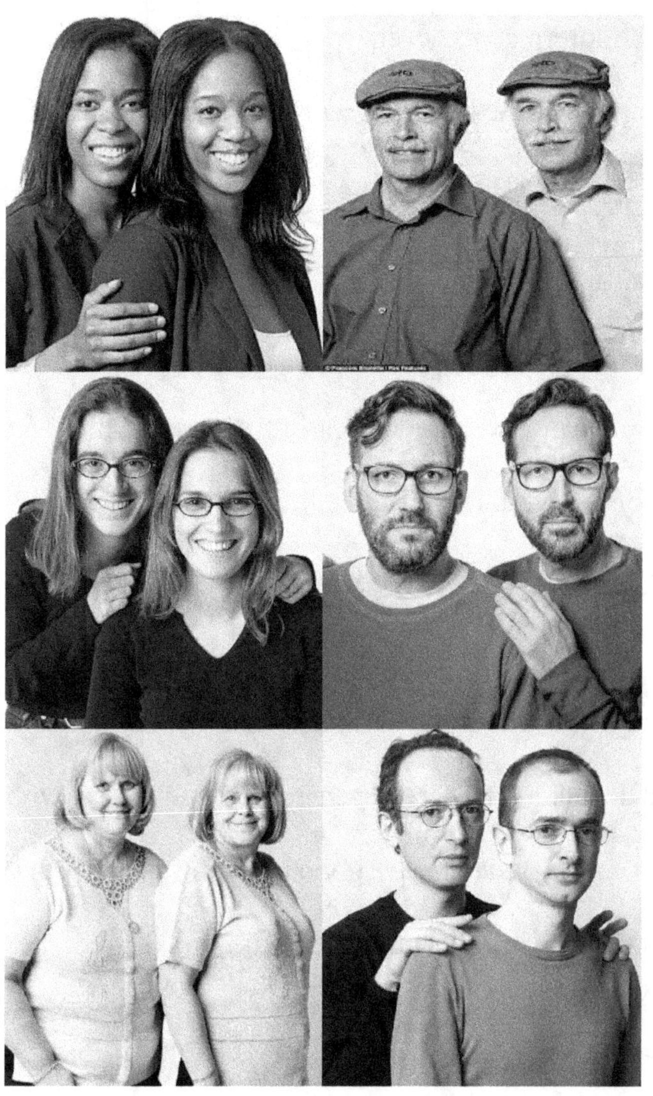

Series "I'm Not a Look-Alike" started in 1999 by photographer François Brunelle

33

This fact becomes more realistic every year due to the increasing human population, which is expected to reach 10 billion inhabitants by the year 2050.

For those with autism spectrum disorder, the situation is similar in the psychological aspect, as it has been shown that people with Asperger's syndrome can have similarities in their personality and even in their way of thinking. For example, it is known that patients diagnosed with Asperger's tend to be loyal, kind, rarely judgmental, find it difficult to gauge their words and expressions, have a relatively childlike spirit, are prone to anxiety and depression, and even find it hard to take offense. In general, an individual with Asperger's is often considered to have a good heart and a loyalty that is hardly matched by a neurotypical person.

# Chapter 6: The Difference Between Tolerance and Inclusion

*"They say that people with Asperger's syndrome are not empathetic... Have you ever put yourself in their place? Do not fear people with autism; embrace them. Do not bother them; simply do not deny them acceptance. Then their abilities will shine because the best gift you can give to someone with ASD is your acceptance and inclusion."*

Tolerance and inclusion are two terms often used together, but they have different meanings. Tolerance refers to the attitude of respecting others' opinions, practices, religions, or even behaviors, even if they differ from one's own. It does not require one to approve of or share those opinions or practices, but simply to accept and not condemn them. Inclusion, on the other hand, refers to a way of treating others that ensures everyone has access to the same rights, resources, and opportunities. Therefore, inclusion is a much more active and equitable concept than tolerance.

In relation to society, tolerance and inclusion function to promote diversity, equality, and respect for individuality. A society where people strive to understand and accept the differentiating traits of others is a society where tolerance reigns; however, this does not necessarily mean the absence of existing prejudices in society, but rather the presence of acceptance of diversity. Inclusion goes a step beyond tolerance, as it not only involves accepting diversity but also recognizing equal opportunities for all. This means that each individual should be treated with the same respect and opportunities, regardless of their religion, race, ethnicity, gender, etc.

That said, there is a theory that claims human behaviors are statistically similar across different people and situations. This theory is based on the hypothesis that, although individuals may have different levels of ability, motivation, and other factors, their short-term actions are the same when placed in similar situations. This theory is called "equidistribution" and is related to the idea of equal opportunity, which is the notion that all human beings have the same right to quality education, employment, and healthcare services regardless of race, sex, religion, disability, orientation, or national origin. This idea emphasizes that we are all human and should be treated equally, regardless of our background. This theory serves as a framework for developing equity and justice in the social sphere and is crucial for preventing discrimination.

The exclusion or even discrimination of autistic individuals can be a discouraging and serious reality. Many autistic people feel excluded by those they share spaces with, whether they are classmates, neighbors, teachers, colleagues, or even loved ones. This happens because many people simply do not understand the life experiences of autistic individuals. This results in a lack of acceptance by others and can lead these individuals to feel isolated and marginalized, which very often triggers symptoms of depression, anger, hatred, and even suicidal tendencies.

According to scientific studies, nearly 66% of people with Asperger's syndrome have considered taking their own lives, while 35% have made specific plans or attempts at suicide or, in the worst cases, have succeeded in taking their lives.

Exclusion can manifest in many ways. People with autism may find that their peers refuse to interact with them, that they are not invited to social gatherings, or that they are even excluded from sports activities. This can be especially terrifying for children trying to socialize with other children at school, as each rejection or exclusion is another blow to their self-esteem.

Adults also often face exclusion. A particularly painful form of this is when an employer decides not to hire a person with autism, or chooses not to promote them or even fires them. Other less obvious forms of exclusion occur in family or social gatherings where the person with autism is not seen as an equal, leading to them being completely ignored or sent to a place where they do not have to socialize with others, causing the affected person a sense of unjustified loneliness and isolation.

The best way to address the exclusion of people with autism is to expand the general understanding of what it means to have autism and any of its spectrums. To solve a problem, we must first understand and accept that we have one. Support and accompaniment can be crucial in helping community members better understand and accept people with autism. As society becomes more informed, we will continue to see greater inclusion and acceptance of autistic people.

Inclusion is not only about involving them in social practices or being kind and empathetic towards them. Inclusion can also refer to emphasizing their respective talents and maximizing their potential. Why is this so important? Because it has been shown that it is common for a person with autism or Asperger's syndrome to have characteristics of a gifted person or at least an above-average intelligence, especially in subjects that greatly interest them. This is due to their greater acuity in information processing compared to the average person. They have better visual memory, a greater capacity to make connections between different elements of a situation, and an innate ability to see details. These abilities allow them to process a much larger amount of information than average, enabling them to gather information and form opinions more quickly.

Some examples of people diagnosed with autism or Asperger's syndrome who had the opportunity to maximize their capacities are historical figures such as the German "Albert Einstein," considered the father of mathematics. Despite having Asperger's syndrome, he revolutionized the world with his mathematical skills and theories on relativity and time travel. We also find Nikola Tesla, the most important inventor of the 20th century, a scientist born in Croatia who more than 100 years ago had already invented objects that we are only beginning to use today, such as drones, wireless energy, alternating current motors, robots, among other things.

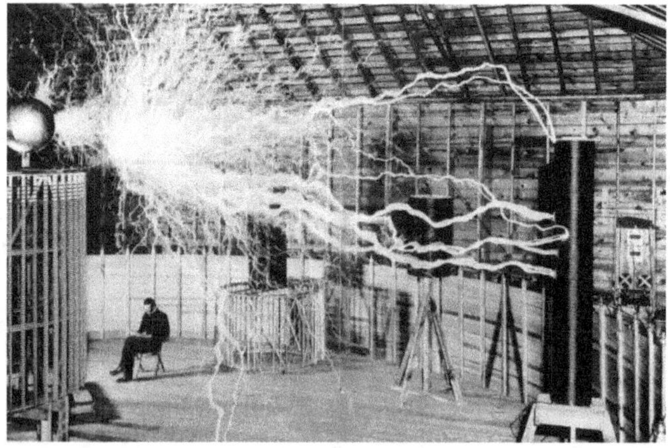

Nikola Tesla with one of his most important inventions: The Tesla coil, created in 1920.

Another person to mention is Temple Grandin, a famous author and university professor born in the United States. She has written numerous books on autism and invented a device to calm cattle, as well as various livestock systems that have been replicated worldwide.

There is also one of the most famous figures of today, South African Elon Musk, who is considered one of the most important entrepreneurs of the 21st century thanks to his various technology companies such as Tesla (electric and autonomous car company), Starlink (unique satellite internet), Neuralink (company aiming to transform the human mind into a tool for controlling objects remotely), and SpaceX (company seeking to take humans to the neighboring planet Mars).

He also became the richest man in the world. Additionally, there are historical figures suspected of having Asperger's or autism, though it cannot be confirmed as we do not know their actual behavior, such as Leonardo Da Vinci, Isaac Newton, and classical music geniuses like Wolfgang Amadeus Mozart and Ludwig van Beethoven.

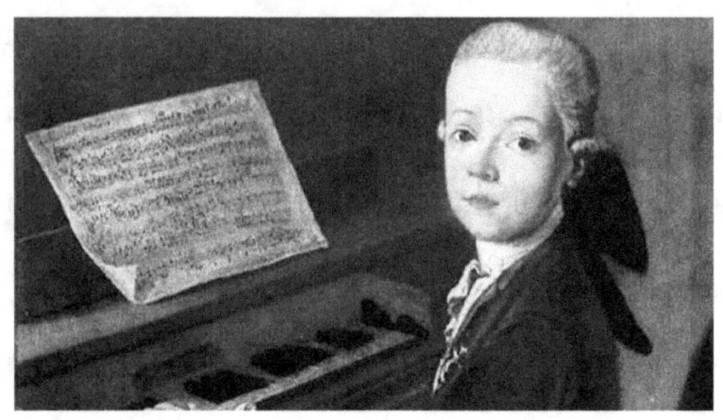

Mozart during the composition of a new sonata.

An interesting fact about Mozart is that his obsessive and repetitive behavior was reflected in his dedication of long hours to music, showing deep concentration and resistance to distractions. He followed specific patterns in his creative process and any interruption bothered him considerably. From a young age, he showed an exceptional interest and ability in music, typical characteristics of Asperger's. Although socially active, he was often considered eccentric and had trouble adapting to social norms. Additionally, he had a keen sensitivity to certain sounds, which could have influenced his unique musical ability. These aspects suggest how Asperger's characteristics may have influenced both the challenges and the extraordinary musical abilities of Mozart.

# Chapter 7: Life with Asperger's

*"And since he didn't know it was impossible... he did it."* To understand Asperger's, you don't need words or formulas, just love. Life with Asperger's is a gift that only those who understand it can appreciate.

Living with Asperger's can be quite difficult for those who have it, as it involves more than just the challenge of making eye contact or the inability to communicate with others as easily as a neurotypical person. Other factors come into play, such as rights, pain, sensitivity to colors, light, and sounds, difficulty recognizing faces, constant distractions, among other things.

Regarding the rights of a person with Asperger's, there are states or entire countries that limit or even prohibit the right to drive for individuals with this disorder. Several arguments are made to justify the prohibition of driving for people with Asperger's. Firstly, there is a concern about their ability to follow traffic rules. People with

ASD may have difficulty interpreting traffic signals, understanding traffic rules, and making decisions in stressful situations.

Another argument is the inability of people with Asperger's to foresee and respond to emergency situations on the road. These situations can include accidents or road problems, and without the ability to interpret situations effectively, it is considered that these individuals could trigger dangerous situations.

A third argument is the concern that people with autism may be too obstinate to heed the advice of road safety experts. This can be dangerous, as the safety of other drivers on the road could be at risk.

Despite these arguments, there is a defense group that argues that people with Asperger's should be allowed to drive, provided they are given the appropriate resources and support. They assert that these individuals have the ability to learn and adapt to traffic rules, and can be ensured safe driving.

Another point is how pain or even emotional distress is interpreted in a person with ASD compared to a neurotypical person. To begin with, people with Asperger's may have a higher sensitivity to external stimuli. They may be more sensitive to sound, light, and touch, which can trigger intense physical and emotional reactions.

For example, a loud sound may be perceived by a person with this disorder as painful or unbearable, resulting in a strong and disturbing reaction just as a very repetitive sound can confuse, irritate, distract, or even exhaust these individuals because such sounds can cause sensory overloads that can seriously affect their information processing capacity.

Furthermore, individuals with ASD have difficulties managing and expressing their emotions. They may feel intense emotions more frequently but may struggle to understand the cause and effect of these emotions in relation to the events they are experiencing. This can result in these individuals experiencing more intense emotional pain than a neurotypical person, as they may feel overwhelmed and distressed without a clear understanding of what is happening.

Likewise, people with Asperger's may experience social pain. Due to their difficulties in interpreting social norms and communicating effectively, they may experience anxiety and stress in social situations. This can result in emotional pain and chronic stress, leading to a decrease in quality of life.

Additionally, these individuals may have difficulties receiving and accepting emotional support from others. They may struggle to communicate their emotional needs and may be less likely to seek help during times of pain and distress. This can result in increased pain and emotional anguish, as they are not receiving the support they need.

On the other hand, people with this disorder can be more sensitive to colors. They may perceive bright, saturated, and contrasting colors with greater intensity. Light can also be a very strong stimulus for them, meaning environments with intense and vibrant lighting can be painful for their nervous system. The exaggerated perception of colors can also impact their mood, as it may inhibit their ability to relax and concentrate.

Finally, and importantly, a person with autism is much more likely to have facial blindness, or "prosopagnosia." Most people recognize faces through a series of cognitive processes that occur in the brain. These processes include visual perception, analysis of individual facial features such as the shape of the nose, the size of the eyes, and the shape of the mouth, analysis of dynamic features like facial expression, and memorization of facial patterns. Researchers believe that individuals with Asperger's Syndrome have difficulties in some of these areas of cognitive processing, resulting in challenges recognizing faces.

One of the most common theories is that these individuals have difficulty processing and retaining visual information due to dysfunction in the temporal lobe of the brain, which is responsible for visual perception. As a result, people with Asperger's Syndrome may struggle to process the facial details necessary to recognize a face. Another theory suggests that these individuals have difficulty recognizing emotion in faces due to dysfunction in the frontal lobe of the brain, which is responsible for emotional processing. This difficulty can make it challenging for them to recognize the faces of people they have met previously.

Additionally, people with ASD may have difficulty processing social information from faces, which can affect their ability to remember and recognize faces. For example, they may struggle to read social cues on a face, making it harder to identify a person.

# Chapter 8: What to Do in an Autistic Crisis

*"It's not about being perfect, it's about being perfectly you."* Bob Marley. *"We don't need to think alike to love alike."* Francis David.

Before discussing an autistic meltdown, we first need to understand exactly what an autistic meltdown is. The term "autistic meltdown" or "autism spectrum meltdown" refers to when a person diagnosed with ASD experiences an intense and overwhelming reaction to specific stimuli or situations. These meltdowns can vary in nature and severity, but they often involve emotional and behavioral difficulties that can be challenging for the individual and those around them. These meltdowns manifest differently depending on the person; some may display behaviors similar to a child having a tantrum, others may scream and self-harm, some may cry while trying to protect themselves from the world, and others might scream and cry while having difficulty breathing. When the individual exhibits such behavior, the correct actions to take are as follows:

- **Keep calm:** The first and most important thing is to remain calm. While a meltdown can be intense and challenging, it's crucial not to panic. A calm and composed demeanor can help the person feel safer.

- **Reduce stimuli:** Identify and eliminate or reduce the stimuli that may be contributing to the meltdown. This could include loud noises, bright lights, crowds, or anything causing sensory overload.

- **Provide a safe environment:** Ensure the environment is safe and free of hazards. Some individuals with ASD may become self-injurious during a meltdown, so it's important to prevent any injuries.

- **Communication:** Try to communicate calmly and understandingly, but avoid asking too many questions or giving complicated instructions. It can be helpful to offer supportive words and remind the person that you are there to help.

- **Know individual needs:** Each person with ASD is unique, and what may calm one person may not work for another. If you know the person and their specific needs, try to tailor your approach accordingly.

- **Use visual language and communication:** Some individuals with ASD may have difficulty with verbal communication during a meltdown. Try using visual communication, such as pictures or gestures, if it helps.

- **Respect personal space:** Respect the person's personal space. It may be helpful to keep a certain distance if the person feels uncomfortable with physical contact.

- **Know the warning signs:** If you know the person and the signs that indicate they are about to have a meltdown, you can intervene before the situation escalates. It can be helpful to develop a prevention plan with the person and their caregivers if possible.

- **Offer emotional support afterward:** After the meltdown has passed, offer emotional support. The person may feel exhausted or overwhelmed, so a calm and understanding environment can be beneficial.

- **Seek professional help:** If the meltdowns are severe or recurrent, it's important to seek help from a healthcare professional or a therapist specialized in ASD. They can provide strategies and therapies to address meltdowns and the specific needs of the person with ASD.

Now, on the other hand: What if you are the patient diagnosed with ASD and you have to deal with a meltdown with no one to help you?

Here are some tips on how to act during an autistic meltdown if you are the person with autism and have no one to help you:

- **Find a safe place:** Look for a quiet and safe place where you can be alone and reduce sensory stimulation. This could be a quiet room, a cozy corner, or any place where you feel safe.
- **Practice breathing techniques:** Try to control your breathing. Inhale deeply through your nose, hold the air for

a few seconds, and then exhale slowly through your mouth. This can help you calm down and reduce anxiety.

- **Use comfort objects:** If you have objects that comfort you, such as a soft blanket, a stress ball, or headphones with relaxing music, use them to help you calm down.

- **Engage in sensory activities:** Some people find it helpful to engage in activities that provide sensory stimulation. This could include squeezing a stress ball, gently rocking, or using a weighted blanket.

- **Internal communication:** Talk to yourself in a soothing manner. Remind yourself that you are safe and that the meltdown will pass. Use self-affirming and supportive phrases.

- **Write or draw:** If it helps, try writing down your thoughts or drawing what you feel. This can be a way to release emotions and process what you are experiencing.

- **Stick to a routine:** If you have an established routine that helps calm you, try to follow it. The familiarity of a routine can provide a sense of security and control.

- **Practice meditation or mindfulness:** If you are familiar with meditation or mindfulness techniques, use them to focus on the present moment and calm your mind.

- **Avoid triggers:** If possible, remove yourself from the situations or stimuli that triggered the meltdown. Avoiding these triggers can help reduce the intensity of the meltdown.

- **Seek professional help:** If you experience frequent meltdowns and find it difficult to manage them on your own, consider seeking the help of a mental health professional or a therapist specializing in autism. They can provide you with additional strategies and tools to handle meltdowns.

Living with autism can sometimes feel overwhelming, but I want you to know that you are not alone. You possess incredible strengths and unique abilities that make you who you are. Each day, you grow stronger, learn more about yourself, and find new ways to navigate this world.

Your perspective is invaluable, and your contributions to society are important. Embrace your uniqueness, celebrate your successes, and be kind to yourself during difficult moments. When you face a crisis, take a moment to find your calm and use the strategies that work best for you. It's okay to ask for help and seek support when you need it.

Believe in your potential. Your talents, creativity, and resilience can shine brightly even in the toughest times. You have the power to overcome obstacles and achieve great things. Trust in your abilities and continue to pursue your passions.

Remember, it's not about being perfect; it's about being perfectly you. Keep moving forward, and know that every step you take is a step toward a brighter future. You are capable, you are strong, and you are worthy of love and acceptance just as you are.

You have a beautiful mind and a unique way of seeing the world. Your journey may be different, but it is filled with limitless possibilities. Keep shining, keep striving, and never forget how extraordinary you are.

Remember, always become the best version of yourself. Do it for yourself and by yourself. **YOU CAN DO IT!**

# Chapter 9: Feeling Whole While Being Alone

*Someone drew a circle to leave me out; however, I made a bigger one to include everyone. There are many ways to be disabled. The most dangerous one is "having no heart."*

When we talk about Asperger's, we automatically talk about loneliness. Why? Because having friends or even a partner can be very complicated for someone with Asperger's, and in extreme cases, even impossible. This initially stems from the difficulty in interacting with others, not knowing how to properly express one's own feelings, and having "uncommon" behaviors that a neurotypical person would never exhibit. Another reason why someone with Asperger's often finds themselves alone is because they develop a self-defense mechanism where they may become asocial or even antisocial to avoid being hurt by others again.

As discussed earlier in this book, a person with Asperger's not only struggles with social interaction but also cannot understand sarcasm, double meanings, non-verbal communication, social protocols, or, in a way, others' feelings. This makes it hard for them to know how to please others and be considered "friends." While it might be easy for someone with Asperger's to see others as friends, there is a possibility that their counterparts are simply being polite and consider them acquaintances or just school or workmates.

Given this, a person with Asperger's may decide to distance themselves from others because a neurotypical person can be selfish by not considering others' feelings or thoughts. What do we mean by this? Let's consider the following example:

Imagine we have a group of five students, including Juan (a patient diagnosed with Asperger's Syndrome). They are all talking and laughing during recess. At one point, Juan decides to make a brief comment, which is not funny to his group of classmates (a group he considers his friends), creating an awkward silence among them. The silence ends when another classmate makes a comment that pleases everyone, and they all laugh and continue talking. This behavior confuses Juan, leading him to wonder if his presence is not welcomed by his friends and classmates or if his comment was distasteful to his peers, making them unwilling to continue the conversation with him.

This forces him to conduct a brief test to see if his presence is welcomed within the group, which involves leaving and announcing his departure to his classmates, hoping to receive responses like "No, stay with us," "Well, we'll go with you later," or "We'll go with you." Clearly, he does not receive these responses; instead, his classmates just briefly say goodbye and continue talking and laughing among themselves. This attitude discourages Juan and we could even say it hurts him, so he withdraws to a solitary place to think about how to start a conversation that might be more pleasing to others.

To help a person with Asperger's feel included in a social group, it's essential first to find common interests, then ask them various questions and have conversations about those questions to foster a bond and a trust area between both parties. It also helps a lot to explain the meanings of certain jokes, words, acronyms, or double-meaning conversations, though the best approach is to strive for the most neutral communication possible.

On the other hand, focusing on the subject of loneliness, solitude can be something that a person with autism might find pleasant depending on the situation or, in some cases, necessary to reorganize thoughts or feel at peace. There is a parable that dates back centuries called "The Two Wolves," which speaks of how within all of us, there are two wolves; one wolf represents anger, resentment, sadness, ego, arrogance, depression, hatred, and pessimism, while the other wolf represents serenity, forgiveness, happiness, companionship, mercy, love, and hope. Both wolves are in a constant struggle, and the only way to know which one will win is depending on which wolf we decide to feed.

For someone with Asperger's, loneliness and exclusion are very common in their lives, which makes them the most resilient and optimistic people compared to a neurotypical person. They always seek to feed the right wolf, continuing their fight for a better life both socially and personally. It's difficult to offend someone with Asperger's because they have managed to accept who they are, as well as their strengths and weaknesses, so from them, we can learn to hold our heads high and achieve our goals despite the mockery and criticism we may receive from society.

In the end, it is possible to be happy alone. Happiness does not depend on others but on oneself. This means that happiness can be found in the present moment, regardless of whether we are alone or accompanied. For each person, the concept of happiness and success is different, but in most cases, for someone with Asperger's, it will always be tied to hope and love.

# Chapter 10: Cure it? Treat it? Control it? NO...understand it.

*"Look, I know I sometimes say or post strange things, but that's just how my brain works. To anyone I've offended, I just want to say: I've reinvented electric cars and I'm sending people to Mars on a rocket, did you think I was going to be a normal, chill guy?" Elon Musk – Diagnosed with ASD.*

Let me tell you a little story: Once, the son of a well-known couple had Asperger's syndrome. In his class, the other kids often made fun of him and excluded him. One day, the boy's father came to the school to talk to his classmates about Asperger's syndrome. He explained that his son was much more than just a different kid; he was a person with a unique gift. He urged them to be more patient and kind with him and to treat him as an equal. He was surprised to see that the other kids started to approach his son. The boy changed a lot since then, socializing with his peers and learning a lot, and his experience helped improve the lives of his class and everyone who knew the boy.

It may seem illogical to some people, but in the past, the treatment of autism was very different from today. In the 1950s, autism treatment focused on re-educating patient behavior, aiming to prevent the development of undesirable behaviors. This included things like implementing strict rules and using punishments to discourage inappropriate behaviors. The treatment also involved addressing behavior with targeted activities, such as using a journal to identify and control inappropriate behaviors.

Another way autism was treated in the past was the use of psychiatric drugs. This included the use of antipsychotics, like phenothiazine, to treat autism symptoms. These medications were thought to help patients calm down and control agitation, anxiety, and other symptoms faced by autistic patients. However, the medications also had numerous side effects that could affect those who took them for life. Currently, these medications are banned because even today, the possible long-term effects on patients are unknown.

In the late 1990s, evidence-based behavioral therapies began to be developed to treat autism. These therapies included Applied Behavior Analysis (ABA) and Applied Language Therapy (ALA). These therapies focus on improving behavior through training, reinforcement, communication, and the use of structure to help patients improve their social, communicative, and self-management skills. These therapies are more widely discussed today and are considered effective treatments for autism.

Now focusing on the topic of understanding, you, the readers, might ask: Why be empathetic and try to adapt to those diagnosed with ASD? Answering your question, we can use the example of the famous historical and current figures mentioned in previous chapters like Isaac Newton, Albert Einstein, or even Elon Musk; all of them had a similarity, that similarity was that they could see details and aspects that no one else managed to see and/or understand.

One of the gifts of a person with ASD or Asperger's is their attention to detail, as they have an exceptional ability to focus on details. This focus can be beneficial in fields such as science, mathematics, medicine, computer science, and engineering, where meticulous attention to detail is essential. We might see some examples of this meticulous attention to detail from these patients in TV series like "The Good Doctor" or documentary films like "Temple Grandin."

Another gift is their outstanding memory; many people with ASD have an exceptional memory for specific facts and details. This can be an asset in fields where precise information retention is crucial, such as history, literature, music, or programming. From this, another gift emerges, which is logical and analytical thinking. Being very literal, patients with ASD can see patterns and connections that others might overlook, which is valuable in disciplines that require problem-solving, such as sciences and research.

Another advantage is creativity and innovation. By paying attention to small details, patients can develop various alternatives and solutions to problems even if they require greater mental planning. This works because an ASD individual can repeat the same situation an incalculable number of times to review all possible scenarios and thus arrive at the best option. The greatest advantage of this gift is that, in most patients, these situations can be reviewed mentally whether they are asleep or awake. In other words, an ASD person can solve an equation, learn a skill, or resolve a conflict through analysis within their dreams.

Another point is that, being very literal, a patient with ASD tends to be very honest, even if it means revealing the harsh truth about things. This can cause potential conflicts and discomfort with those who do not yet have an understanding and tolerance towards these patients. Another conflict is that, due to their honesty and lack of filters, patients with ASD might say things that could make people in the same room uncomfortable. Some examples could be: *"I would like to dress up as a dinosaur for Halloween because I love dinosaurs and I once thought about acting like one." "I need to know how to pamper my girlfriend on our anniversary because many say the right thing to do is to have sex, although we have never practiced it." "I would like to talk to my dog to better understand its needs; I hope they make a dog translator soon."*

On the other hand, honesty can also work in favor of the patients because if others understand the ASD situation, they can be great company. A bond of trust and transparency develops between both parties, leaving behind hypocrisy, lack of trust, and even those little lies that could harm any of the parties involved in the long run.

The last gift that can be considered in ASD and Asperger's patients is their deep empathy, kindness, tolerance, and love towards others. While it is true that people with this disorder have difficulty understanding human emotions (which has often led them to be associated as non-empathetic individuals), it is also true that patients can demonstrate empathy in their own way.

Let's take an example: An Asperger's high school student is being attacked by his theater classmates because he offended his classmate by saying that due to her physique and skin color, she doesn't look anything like the actress Gal Gadot. The patient cannot understand why his comment is offensive to his classmates, since analytically and literally speaking, his classmate is dark-skinned, relatively short in stature, and has a slightly elevated body mass index for her age.

On the other hand, what would happen if the situation involved a new girl that no one wants to talk to, and therefore she feels lonely? Most likely, the patient would seek to interact with her and make her feel better about herself. This empathy and sensitivity to what they might call injustice and lack of collective empathy arise mainly from the experiences the patient has had to deal with. Because of this sensitivity, they feel morally compelled to be active defenders of causes they consider important. Another advantage is the tolerance and kindness that patients with ASD can boast, as their individual experiences make them very understanding, kind, and tolerant toward other people regardless of their orientation, gender, disability, beliefs, race, or economic situation.

Despite everything, it is possible that the greatest advantage of an Asperger and generally any person with ASD is the incredible loyalty, love, and unconditional support they can give to those they consider their friends and/or family. This is because these patients find it very difficult to socialize and even more difficult to form bonds of love or friendship with neurotypicals. Therefore, when they find a partner or a friend, they will do their best to care for them and keep them close. It is possible that the biggest mistake of an Asperger is thinking they have many friends just because their work or schoolmates were kind to them, exchanged conversations, or are friends on social media.

Like a child finding out that Santa Claus doesn't exist, patients may experience depression and anxiety when they realize that despite thinking in the past that everyone was their friend, very few people actually consider them a friend or, in the worst case, they realize that they really don't have any friends.

This can be difficult to assimilate for the affected person because before understanding the harsh reality, they had already felt affection and some attachment towards their peers, thinking that they would also have the same attachment or way of thinking towards them.

That said, these are the main reasons to understand and empathize with a person with ASD. In the end, it is possible that, upon closer inspection, a person with autism has more empathy towards others than a neurotypical person simply because neurotypical people think more about themselves than others, whether voluntarily or involuntarily.

**INTERVIEW #1**

**What is your name?**

My name is Salvador and I am 24 years old.

**Do you consider yourself different from those around you? Why?**

Yes. Since I was a child, I considered myself different, although it was hard to understand why. I thought this was normal since everyone is unique, but I had more noticeable traits than others. For example, not understanding hints, metaphors, or local expressions. Over time, I have understood them better, but even today, I sometimes struggle to understand things that aren't literal. My accent is also something that stands out because whenever I meet someone, they usually ask where I am from due to my accent. Later, I learned that this is a common aspect for people with Asperger's (Autism Spectrum Disorder) and it is called a "monotone accent." Another thing would be my hearing; I hear noises louder than others. I have worked in factories, and the ambient noises in those places overwhelm me a lot. Although I have gotten used to it over time, there are days when I simply can't stand them and suffer internally. This aspect has affected me socially since ambient noises easily drown out voices for me, and people think I'm deaf or not paying attention. I ask them to repeat what they said, but sometimes I still can't hear them well. Out of embarrassment and to keep the conversation flowing, I have to continue listening despite not understanding the "drowned out" words, which makes me miss parts of the conversation and have to pretend I heard everything to avoid embarrassment and the annoyance of the person speaking to me.

**When did you find out you had Asperger's? How did you find out, and what was your reaction upon learning?**

I found out at 15 years old. I didn't see it as a big deal since I told the people close to me and decided to resume my therapy. I had been going to special therapy as a child, but for some reason, my parents stopped taking me at some point.

**Can you tell us a bit about Asperger's in your own words? Do you consider it important for people to know about this disorder?**

Personally, I consider the disorder something that makes you a little different, making you attentive in a work setting but affecting you somewhat socially. It is very important for everyone to know about Asperger's (ASD). The few people I have met who know about it are already parents, which makes me happy because they are aware that their children might have it. However, on the other hand, the rest have never heard of it in their lives. I feel it is important to know about it, whether people want to be parents or not, so that a better environment can be created for everyone.

**What was/is your life like in school/university?**

Chaotic. Although in the early years of primary school, subjects seemed very simple to me, as time went on and they became more complex, I lost interest. Considering that people with Asperger's (ASD) tend to be good and obsessive in areas they like and only in those areas, subjects weren't among the things I enjoyed. I preferred drawing, music, and a bit of learning English. The rest didn't matter much to me, and I had a very hard time studying. Things got worse between primary and secondary school. Besides going through a rough time that led to a depression I still deal with today, it only worsened my school performance, with little interest in social and academic matters. Finally, in high school, which I didn't finish due to financial situation and my declining interest, I lost all interest in finishing my studies. Nowadays, I am not at all interested in completing my education and would prefer to focus academically on my interests.

**Did you ever talk about your disorder with your teachers and/or classmates? If so, how did they react?**

I wasn't very open about it back then when I found out and was in high school. However, over time and on the advice of my psychologist, I try to talk about it with my work colleagues, and their reaction is usually one of amazement, either because they don't know about the disorder or because they do know and suspected it due to my behavior.

**Do you prefer solitude or being with other people?**

Being alone gives me the few moments of peace I have during the day, although I often prefer to be with the people I care about just as much. However, I hate being surrounded by strangers or people I really don't like, as it gives me a feeling of stress compared to when I am alone.

**What are your biggest difficulties being Asperger's?**

Mostly social. I developed a very introverted behavior to the point where I can spend hours or even the whole day without interacting with a single person since I usually don't talk to anyone until they talk to me first. Besides the hearing issue I mentioned earlier, which has affected me socially and personally, as people, even knowing my condition, get annoyed thinking that I am ignoring them when I ask them to repeat words I didn't hear well.

**What are your biggest interests and dreams for the future?**

Due to my depression, I lost interest in the future and knowing what I want in life. However, I prefer to continue with my interests, such as music and drawing, even as a hobby, since I will give my greatest interest in work without anything to highlight, comfortable in the few activities I can do well, such as repetitive jobs without much complexity, to continue living as an adult without many motivations in life.

**Do you have friends and/or a partner? Can you tell me a story about how they came to be in your life?**

I have one friend. He's quite active and a bit of a mess. I met him in high school, but I didn't talk to him until the second semester because we shared the same interest in music, and there wasn't really any other reason. After high school, he was the only one of my classmates I saw more often throughout my journey, either because we ended up at the same high school or because I occasionally ran into him on the street. Since then, we've shared more interests like video games, TV shows, or food, and without realizing it, he gradually became my best friend. He never paid attention to or judged me for who I am; he just wanted the best for me, and we started getting closer in our work, either by giving him advice or him giving me advice.

**If you were ever told that there is a possibility of becoming neurotypical and leaving Asperger's behind, would you accept leaving Asperger's? Why?**

I would accept it. Being Asperger's has brought me good things, like performance at work or being organized, but on the other hand, it has made me feel very bad about myself, as I have never been able to socialize well or perform better in school or other areas of life, and that led to my depression.

**Are you proud of who you are as a person? What do you consider your purpose in life?**

Honestly, I don't know. In some things, I feel good about myself, even proud of being able to carry out a double mental effort to lead a normal adult life. But on the other hand, I feel that I can't meet the expectations to have the life I want, alongside someone I love, and I feel that I will never be up to the level of a functional person. Honestly, I consider myself to have no purpose, just another pedestrian on the road, only serving society and that's it.

**Do you have any message to give to your future readers? And to your future self?**

I wish you all the best in the world. Despite giving an impression of myself that is somewhat unmotivating, I feel it is a necessary point of view for those parents with Asperger's children, to see a reflection of their children's future if they do not take their disorder into account, and what can lead to bad decisions, as well as other adults with Asperger's. You are not alone. Take that step towards therapy; it's never too late. Despite having mental scars, they can still be treated and have a more pleasant life, even if you don't have anyone's support. I want to tell you that it is possible.

**INTERVIEW #2**

**What is your name?**

Good day, my name is Sebastián and I am 21 years old.

**Do you consider yourself different from those around you? Why?**

Yes, I have always considered myself different from others. When I was a child, I barely noticed it because it was easier for me to forget social problems or what other kids said about me when I was with my friends. In high school, there were moments when I thought I was different from others because I had a superior mind or simply because I didn't blindly follow trends. At that time, I didn't understand that being "weird" to others or simply different to my family was more focused on a disorder and not so much on intellect.

**When did you find out you had Asperger's? How did you find out and what was your reaction when you knew?**

I found out I had Asperger's at the age of 13 during therapy sessions with a psychologist because the bullying in my high school was getting worse, and I felt increasingly depressed. When they explained to me that I had Asperger's syndrome, I personally felt free to finally understand that those around me didn't have a problem with me or my personality, but that I had a mental disorder that made me see, hear, and experience the world differently from others. It wasn't tolerated primarily due to a lack of empathy from others and secondly due to a lack of information about it.

**Can you tell us a little about Asperger's in your own words? Do you think it is important for people to know about this disorder?**

For me, Asperger's is a mental disorder that we are born with and makes us feel, see, and hear the world in a completely different way from a neurotypical person. It is something that, although it can give us both advantages and disadvantages, gives us our essence of who we are as people. I consider it very important for people to truly understand what this disorder entails and that, no matter how much you try, it is not something that has a cure or treatment. People usually show selfish or unempathetic behavior towards mental disorders, thinking that things just go away simply by wanting it or by taking medication. Another point is that it is important for them to learn that there are tens of millions of people worldwide with this disorder, and as far as I know, the number increases year by year, either due to inheritance or some other unknown cause.

**How was/is your life in school/university?**

Honestly, my life back then was a mess. While I had good moments, I also had too many bad moments to the point where I currently want to forget certain stages of my life. In fact, I started going to a psychologist in high school because the bullying I suffered every day was affecting me more and more. It wasn't the typical physical bullying, but verbal. They also tended to ignore me for being "weird," and even the teachers, instead of helping, always defended my classmates. One thing you learn being Asperger's is that people don't defend those who truly deserve it or are on the right side; they support those they like better, regardless of whether that support affects others. This is true whether you're a child, teenager, or adult. Being Asperger's means being alone in an incomprehensible world where it seems everyone speaks a different language and has a different culture than we are used to, and no matter how much we try to adapt, it is simply impossible for us.

**Did you ever talk about your disorder with your teachers and/or classmates? If so, how did they react?**

I never felt the need to do so because I knew things wouldn't change. It's like trying to explain the string theory scientifically to someone who has only ever learned the name of the theory. If we ask people what Asperger's is to them, they almost always say it's simply autism but less intense. So, how can you explain something they're not interested in learning about? At work, I have explained it to my colleagues; however, despite the results being pretty much as expected, they have learned to tolerate and accept my disorder, though they haven't learned to include it. Personally, I consider that progress.

**Do you prefer solitude or being in the company of others?**

It depends a lot on the situation. In general, I like being alone because I can focus on my own things, and I always like to use headphones and listen to music. On the other hand, if I'm surrounded by people, I don't like feeling alone, so I either go somewhere to be alone or try to join the person I trust the most and see if they like my presence or not to evaluate whether I stay or leave. Even so, in both cases, I think I wouldn't like to be 100% alone if I'm with my best friend.

**What are your biggest difficulties being Asperger's?**

As an Asperger, my biggest difficulties are mainly socializing with other people since part of socializing is knowing how to make jokes and have long conversations with people. This is very difficult for us because not understanding sarcasm or double meanings makes it hard for us to know when someone is joking or telling a joke. We also can't have long conversations if the other person isn't the one initiating and continuing the conversation because it's almost impossible for us to start and proceed with conversations, especially if they're not about the topic we like the most.

Another point that affected me a lot in school was attention deficit because, although I am a very intelligent person, it wasn't reflected in my grades, especially in exams.

Another thing is eye contact. Part of socializing with people is that you always have to look them in the eyes; otherwise, they may consider it rude or think of us as serious and antisocial people when, in reality, it makes us very uncomfortable to look into others' eyes, even if we don't have a specific reason for that discomfort. Still, I have practiced looking into other people's eyes when it comes to work or people I'm just starting to meet, and so far, it has worked well.

**What are your biggest interests and future dreams?**

My biggest interests are architecture, astronomy, and languages. In fact, I always dreamed of being an astronomer, but I never had the geographical or economic opportunities to achieve it. Despite that, I continue to learn about it as a hobby. In the case of languages, I really enjoy learning, so I am currently a polyglot. My future goal is to be a philanthropic politician who, thanks to his knowledge and languages, can be considered the noblest, most intelligent, and philanthropic ruler in the history of my country. Of course, I know it's very difficult to achieve, but if I can leave my mark on this world before I die, I would consider that a personal achievement.

**Do you have friends and/or a partner? Can you tell me a story of how they came to be?**

I have three friends whom I consider my best friends. I met each one at different stages of my life, and although it sounds somewhat illogical, the truth is that they do not resemble me in any social or personality aspect. My best friends are very sociable and have somewhat high egos. They frequently change partners and have very active social lives, so when we first met, we didn't like each other. However, due to fate, we ended up becoming best friends despite not having similar interests or always having something to talk about.

Once, I decided to ask each one why I was their best friend, and each had different versions. One told me it was because he knew that despite everything, I was a loyal and sincere friend. He didn't need to be surrounded by many people if they spoke badly behind his back or if he doubted how much they would be there for him through thick and thin. He not only appreciated my friendship but was also grateful for it.

My second best friend said it was because I was proof that to form a friendship and believe in love of any kind, words are not needed, just always being there even if there were no topics of conversation.

Lastly, my third friend said that despite being surrounded by many friends and always being at gatherings and parties, he appreciated having someone who had no filters or judgments. Someone who had deep and reflective conversations beyond simple sports or party topics. He also liked that when he did things well, I would congratulate him, and when he did things wrong, I would tell him firmly. This made him understand that someone really cared about him, and he knew that I would always seek the best for him as long as it was ethically good or for the greater good of both him and others.

**If you were ever told there was a possibility of becoming neurotypical and leaving Asperger's behind, would you accept to stop being Asperger? Why?**

I would really think about it, but I know the answer would be a resounding no. This is because, although Asperger's has brought me many problems in life (especially social ones), the truth is that it is part of me, it is my essence, it is a symbol that characterizes me as a person, and it represents me as a loyal, noble, neutral, and loving person, even if this cannot be understood by the rest of the people.

**Are you proud of who you are as a person? What do you consider to be your purpose in life?**

Yes, in a way, I am proud of myself, but at the same time, I do not yet feel truly satisfied with who I am because I know that as a person, I still have a long way to go, many goals to achieve, and many dreams to make come true.

**Do you have any message for your future readers? And for your future self?**

My message is that if you are Asperger, I want you to know that you are not alone. There are many of us in the world who have gone through what you have gone through or are even going through now, but I want you to remember that the noblest and most intelligent minds in history also went through the same things we did and never gave up. I don't know, maybe you will become the next Nikola Tesla or Elon Musk or Albert Einstein or Stephen Hawking, but you will never know if you get depressed. Be strong because the future will look at you with better eyes.

## INTERVIEW #3

**What is your name?**

My name is Cristina Hernández and I am a Neurobiologist.

**Do you consider yourself different from those around you? Why?**

Yes, when I didn't have the Asperger's diagnosis, I always thought there was something strange about me, that I didn't fit into society because I had different tastes and interests and even a different way of expressing myself in all aspects compared to my family or classmates. In fact, my parents always knew there was something "not normal" about me, so they took me to various psychologists when I was a child, and each one diagnosed me with all kinds of mental illnesses or even commented that the problem was my lack of nutrition, something that personally didn't make any sense to me.

**When did you find out you had Asperger's? How did you find out and what was your reaction when you knew?**

I was diagnosed very late, more specifically at 18 years old. Until that age, I was depressed due to the taunts and criticisms from my classmates; however, when I found out I had Asperger's, I felt liberated because now I understood what was really happening with me. I no longer felt bad because I began to understand that being different from the rest of society didn't make me bad, just unique.

**Can you tell us a bit about Asperger's in your own words? Do you think it's important for people to know about this disorder?**

For me, Asperger's is a subcategory of the autism spectrum, something you are born with, live with, and die with, so it has neither treatment nor cure. In other words, you are born Asperger and you die Asperger.

**How was/is your life in school/university?**

Personally, I always wanted to forget primary and secondary school. Many people laughed at me because I was "weird"; in fact, I isolated myself to avoid having to endure the torment of being repeatedly told that I was different from the rest. The bullying I suffered might have been a brief stage in my life, but it's something that marks you for life. Even now, I continue to have memories in the form of nightmares from my childhood and adolescence.

Personally, I would be very afraid to go back to school because being surrounded by people my age would remind me of those old times when I had to hide in the most secluded place in the classroom, praying the teacher wouldn't call me to the front. Probably if I hadn't suffered such brutal bullying, despite changing schools and suffering it for almost 17 years, I think I wouldn't be an activist today and wouldn't fight for all the things I fight for now.

**Did you ever talk about your disorder with your teachers and/or classmates? If so, how did they react?**

Not really, I always considered it might be a waste of time because the teachers weren't empathetic and were probably never taught about the various mental disorders a child could suffer from and how to act in each situation. In the case of my classmates, by the time I knew my diagnosis, I was already studying at university, so I mostly spent my time studying and not socializing. In fact, during secondary school, I always told the teachers when my classmates bothered me, but they really didn't do anything.

**Do you prefer solitude or being around other people?**

The truth is, I've always valued being alone, but the reality is that I also think I was alone and enjoyed that solitude because I didn't know how to relate to others. Now that I have truly discovered myself and, with practice, managed to socialize with some people, I am beginning to value being with my boyfriend or my friends. It's true that my moments of solitude have been reduced (and in a way, I miss it), but I think this is a phase in my life where I feel very happy because I am overcoming myself.

**What are your biggest challenges being Asperger?**

I could consider making eye contact as one of them. Of course, not so much now, but as a child, it was very hard for me. One of the things that bothered my father the most about me was that when he scolded me, I wouldn't look him in the eyes. He would say, "Look at me, Cristina," and I would say, "No, I can't." He interpreted that gesture as defiance, so the arguments always lasted longer. For that reason, he never really understood that I genuinely couldn't make eye contact.

**What are your greatest interests and future dreams?**

I don't think I have a specific answer because my interests have changed over time. When I was 6, I read Shakespeare; years later, my interests changed, and I knew the Egyptian gods in alphabetical order and had a mineral collection hidden under my bed. Nowadays, my interests are neurobiology and chemistry, and possibly in the future, I'll have another interest. However, my future dream is to discover precisely the reason for the existence of Asperger's and other autism spectrums.

**Do you have friends and/or a partner? Can you tell me a story about how they became so?**

It's a very funny but long story, so I'll summarize it this way: My husband is also a neurobiologist. Thanks to him, I feel free; I can be the person I've always wanted to be, and I know he will support me at all times. With him, I finally feel liberated. As for friends, it's still hard for me to understand when someone is truly my friend. I don't know the boundary between acquaintance and friend. We handle the concept of "friendship" differently; we really wish that everyone in the world could be friends and that even after months without talking, we know they would still be our friends.

**If you were ever told there was a possibility of becoming neurotypical and leaving Asperger's behind, would you accept to stop being Asperger? Why?**

Personally, I would say no. In my case, I can say that many times I have pretended to be "normal," although I don't really understand what normal is for people because we live in a world where people don't understand us, or we don't understand the world. But I wouldn't accept it because having Asperger's has made me see life through different eyes. For me, it's clear to see and hear birds, but people, despite having a bird in front of them, simply don't really see it. Another thing I like about having Asperger's is that I am a person without filters, so I am not afraid to say or ask anything.

**Are you proud of who you are as a person? What do you consider your purpose in life to be?**

Yes, I am very proud of who I am as a person because despite all the social, family, and even personal conflicts, I managed to move forward with my head held high and became a neurobiologist who day by day fights to know the great questions of the human mind and the functioning of the brain itself.

**Do you have any message to give to your future readers? And to your future self?**

My message is that whether you are Asperger or neurotypical, everything happens for a reason, so don't give up despite any difficulties. We are all unique, and that gives us our own identity, so be proud of yourselves and always fight for what is good, not just for humans but for all organisms in general.

**INTERVIEW #4**

**What is your name?**

My name is Melissa and I am 14 years old.

**Do you consider yourself different from those around you? Why?**

Yes, I feel it might be because I find it difficult to interact properly with others or simply because I don't act the way others do and how I am expected to act by them.

**When did you find out you had Asperger's? How did you find out and what was your reaction when you found out?**

Around the age of 8. I suppose I wasn't very surprised by it because I was already somewhat familiar with what it was since one of my brothers had been previously diagnosed from an early age and it was mentioned sometimes. But when I found out that I had it too, I didn't really think much of it, although it just made sense that I had it given my behavior and way of thinking.

**Can you tell us a little about Asperger's in your own words? Do you think it's important for people to know about this disorder?**

In general, I think being Asperger's means seeing the world from a different perspective than how it's normally seen by others; even thinking, expressing oneself, and feeling differently and reacting to situations differently too. The characteristics can vary in each person since, as it's a spectrum, it might not be the same for everyone. Personally, I would say it's important so that others can understand us better.

**What was/is your life like in school/university?**

I would say it's somewhat boring; I don't enjoy it much. I don't talk much, I'm mostly quiet, and I get nervous being there. Socially, I have some difficulty making friends and talking to others first unless they do, and I tend to avoid interacting with others sometimes. But if they interact with me first, I feel bad if I ignore them, so I don't, but at the same time, it tires me a bit. In terms of studies, I just try my best to get good grades and fulfill whatever is asked of me.

**Have you ever talked about your disorder with your teachers and/or classmates? If so, how did they react?**

I haven't, but my mom has had to do it a few times. After she talked to the teachers, I think they have been understanding about it, although I couldn't say the same for my classmates because despite everything, I continued to be somewhat excluded from social groups.

**Do you prefer solitude or being around other people?**

I prefer solitude; it makes me feel better about myself and gives me more opportunities to focus on my own thoughts.

**What are your biggest difficulties being Asperger's?**

Dealing with people, staying focused all the time, making sure I never do anything that might bother or make others uncomfortable or seem weird (or accidentally say something nonsensical), saying too much without meaning to or without knowing it's unnecessary, and expressing myself to others in a correct and "normal" way.

**What are your biggest interests and future dreams?**

I don't think I have any. I don't think much about it and have no idea what to expect. I prefer to focus on the present rather than the future.

**Do you have friends and/or a partner? Can you tell me a story about how they came to be?**

For now, I've only had friends. Some have been from school who talked to me first, and gradually we started talking more until we became friends, or they simply asked if I wanted to be their friend. But most of my closest friendships have been online; I didn't meet everyone the same way, but the others usually or almost always took the first step to initiate a friendship with me or were the first to start a conversation with me expecting a response from my side.

**If you were ever told there was a possibility to become neurotypical and leave Asperger's behind, would you accept leaving Asperger's? Why?**

I would probably say no because personally, I'm fine being Asperger's; it's part of me after all, which makes me feel more like myself. If I weren't, I would likely be very different, and I think it would be unusual or strange for me.

**Are you proud of who you are as a person? What do you consider your purpose in life?**

I wouldn't say I'm proud of who I am for many reasons, and I don't really know what my purpose in life is. Maybe I'll know in the future considering all my talents, but for now, I'm too young to know.

**Do you have any message for your future readers? And to your future self?**

I would say that there's nothing wrong with being Asperger's. Maybe we are different from others, but that doesn't mean we are less or incapable of what neurotypicals can do. And maybe I would tell my future self that it's okay to be myself and not always be like others because we can achieve things that a normal person would never be able to do.

**INTERVIEW #5**

**What is your name?**

My name is Alexis and I am 17 years old.

**Do you consider yourself different from those around you? Why?**

Yes, because I feel that my way of thinking is different compared to others and that I see the world and situations in a way that a neurotypical person would not be accustomed to.

**When did you find out you had Asperger's? How did you find out and what was your reaction to knowing?**

I found out about 10 years ago when I was in first grade. At that time, I didn't know what Asperger's syndrome or a mental disorder was in general, so I didn't react negatively, although I'm not completely sure because I don't remember much from those years.

**Can you tell us a bit about Asperger's in your own words? Do you consider it important for people to know about this disorder?**

In my personal opinion, I think Asperger's syndrome is a syndrome that could be misunderstood or confused with another disorder by most of the population. Yes, I consider it important for people to be informed about this syndrome for the reasons mentioned above and also because I feel that Asperger's syndrome is not very visible, so to speak, to the general population. Schools don't even teach students about these topics, which I consider a grave mistake, given that it is possible that at least one student may have at least one type of mental disorder, and due to a lack of training, teachers may show really intolerant attitudes towards them.

**What was/is your life like in school/university?**

In primary school, it went very badly. I thought I had friends because I hung out with them, but I didn't understand that they didn't consider me their friend but more of a pawn, as they took advantage of or made fun of me on several occasions, but I didn't understand it at the time. In first grade of secondary school, it wasn't much better, but later I started an exhaustive process to stop making the same mistakes, so after the pandemic, I put my new social and psychological skills into practice in the little time I had left of in-person high school. That made my brief time there one of the happiest of my life, or at least until now. I also plan to use these same skills in university.

**Did you ever talk about your disorder to your teachers and/or schoolmates? If so, how did they react?**

I only told my classmates in primary school, as well as my primary and secondary school teachers. Interestingly, my primary school classmates simply didn't care much. I suppose it's because they found out through a classmate who "discovered" it and told the others, although at this point I wonder if they really understood what the disorder entailed or if they considered it a disease.

**Do you prefer solitude or being in the company of others?**

It depends a lot on the type of people I'm with. I prefer to be in the company of others, but only if it's the right kind of people, like friends or empathetic people. If that's not the case, then I prefer solitude. As the saying goes, it's better to be alone than in bad company.

**What are your biggest difficulties being Asperger's?**

In general, socializing is difficult for me because I find it very hard to understand social protocols, sarcasm, double meanings, and people's non-verbal language. It stresses me out not knowing if someone is saying something seriously or if they're joking or being sarcastic.

**What are your main interests and dreams for the future?**

My interests are very varied. For example, I'm into cars (I have a very complete Hot Wheels collection), technology (such as artificial intelligence, technological advances in all fields, robotics, or just tech gadgets), and of course, video games like anyone my age. As for my dreams for the future, I have many, but I wouldn't know what to say specifically since I'm at a key age to figure out who I want to be in the future.

**Do you have friends and/or a partner? Can you tell me a story about how they came to be?**

Yes, in fact, I could say I have quite a few friends, and I met most of them in secondary and high school, but I can't think of a specific story to tell right now.

**If you were ever told there was a possibility to become neurotypical and leave Asperger's behind, would you accept it? Why?**

I'm not really sure because I'd have to think about it carefully. Nowadays, I feel like my life wouldn't be too different from how it is now, but if that possibility had existed during my childhood and part of my adolescence, I probably would have accepted it.

**Are you proud of who you are as a person? What do you consider your purpose in life to be?**

I don't know what to say about being proud of who I am, and I honestly don't know what my purpose in life is. But I know that the world is not on the right track in many aspects, whether economic, social, psychological, or environmental, so my purpose is the least of my worries.

**Do you have any message for your future readers? And to your future self?**

I'd personally say that Asperger's syndrome shouldn't be an obstacle to being happy or having a normal life. To my future self, I'd say that I hope I've escaped from Latin America. It's an intolerant region with many social problems that I don't want to be a part of, but I hope that one day these will be things of the past and people can live freely and happily for who they are, regardless of their economic, mental, or social situation.

**INTERVIEW #6**

**What is your name?**

My name is Juan, and I am 34 years old.

**Do you consider yourself different from those around you? Why?**

Yes, I consider myself different. My mind works differently; I am usually very meticulous and have very specific interests that I am deeply passionate about. While others may be more sociable and adapt easily to new situations, I prefer structure and routine.

**When did you find out you had Asperger's? How did you find out, and what was your reaction?**

I found out when I was 14 years old. My parents and I noticed that I had difficulties socializing and understanding certain social dynamics, so they decided to seek professional help. A psychologist diagnosed me with Asperger's syndrome. At first, I felt confused and a bit scared, but then it was a relief to understand why I felt different and that there was an explanation for my experiences.

**Can you tell us a bit about Asperger's in your own words? Do you think it's important for people to know about this disorder?**

Sure. For me, Asperger's syndrome is like having a different operating system. My brain processes information differently than most people. I have trouble understanding social cues, and sometimes conversations can be confusing because I don't easily pick up on body language or tone of voice. However, it also allows me to have great focus on my interests, which helps me delve deep and become an expert in those areas.

Yes, I think it's very important for people to know about this disorder. Often, people with Asperger's are misunderstood and labeled as weird or antisocial when in reality they simply experience and perceive the world differently. With more awareness and understanding, people can learn to be more patient and empathetic, making social interactions easier and less stressful for us. Moreover, knowing about Asperger's can help others appreciate the unique skills and perspectives we bring, fostering a more inclusive and enriching environment for everyone.

**How was/is your life in school/university?**

For me, school was really challenging. I didn't like changes in routine, and social interactions exhausted me. I struggled to make friends and often felt lonely. However, I excelled in subjects that interested me, like math and computer science. In university, I found more people with interests similar to mine, and although socializing was still difficult, it was easier to find my place.

**Have you ever talked about your disorder with your teachers and/or schoolmates? If so, how did they react?**

Yes, I talked to some teachers and classmates about my disorder. Most of my teachers were understanding and tried to help me, adapting their teaching methods to my needs when possible. My classmates had mixed reactions; some treated me with more patience, while others didn't understand or didn't care much.

**Do you prefer solitude or being in the company of others?**

I prefer solitude most of the time. Being alone allows me to focus on my interests without the distractions of social interactions. However, I also appreciate the company of a few close people with whom I feel comfortable.

**What are your biggest challenges being Asperger's?**

The biggest challenges include understanding and managing the subtleties of non-verbal communication, dealing with unexpected changes in my routine, and facing sensory overload in noisy or chaotic environments. It's also difficult to explain to others how I feel or why I react a certain way.

**What are your biggest interests and dreams for the future?**

My biggest interests are programming and technology. I dream of developing software that can help improve people's lives, especially those with special needs. I'm not sure what exactly I will do yet, but I'm certain that whatever I do will help others.

**Do you have friends and/or a partner? Can you tell me a story about how they came to be?**

I have a few close friends. I met my best friend in college, in a robotics club. At first, our interactions were limited, but over time, we realized that we shared many interests and ways of thinking. Our friendship grew from there, based on mutual understanding and respect.

**If you were ever told that there was a possibility of becoming neurotypical and leaving Asperger's behind, would you accept leaving Asperger's behind? Why?**

I don't think I would accept. While Asperger's comes with challenges, it has also given me unique skills and a different perspective on the world. It has allowed me to delve deeply into my interests in a way that I believe wouldn't be possible otherwise. I am proud of who I am and how I think.

**Are you proud of who you are as a person? What do you consider your purpose in life?**

Yes, I am proud of who I am. My purpose in life is to use my skills and unique perspective to make a positive contribution to society. I want to help others through technology and advocate for the acceptance and understanding of people with autism spectrum disorders.

**Do you have any message for your future readers? And for your future self?**

To the people who will read this in the future, I would say that everyone has their own value and unique perspective, and it's important to be understanding and patient with others, especially those who think and feel differently. To my future self, I would say to keep being true to yourself and continue pursuing your dreams, no matter the obstacles you may encounter along the way.

**INTERVIEW #7**

**What is your name?**

My name is Diego, and I am 10 years old.

**Do you consider yourself different from those around you? Why?**

Yes, I feel a bit different because I love talking about dogs, and sometimes other kids don't understand why I get so excited. I also like to be alone during recess while the other kids play together.

**When did you find out you had Asperger's? How did you find out, and what was your reaction to knowing?**

My parents and a doctor told me I had Asperger's when I was 7 years old. I didn't understand much at first, but they explained that my brain works a little differently. I felt a bit confused, but then I realized that this explains why some things are more difficult for me than for other kids.

**What is your life like at school?**

At school, I really like natural sciences because they teach us about animals and ecosystems. But sometimes, recess is hard because I don't know how to join in the other kids' games. I also like to sit and read about animals on an e-book that my mom gave me.

**Have you ever talked about your disorder with your teachers and/or schoolmates? If so, how did they react?**

Yes, my mom and I talked to my teacher about my Asperger's. She was very kind and now helps me when I feel overwhelmed. Some classmates don't understand well, but others accept me as I am, and that makes me happy.

**Do you prefer solitude or being in the company of others?**

I prefer to be alone most of the time because I can think and play with my toys without interruptions. But I also like being with my best friend because he understands my interests.

**What are your biggest challenges being Asperger's?**

I find it hard to understand when other kids are joking or when they are angry with me. Loud noises and unexpected changes also bother me a lot and make me feel uncomfortable.

**What are your biggest interests and dreams for the future?**

I love everything related to dogs because I have a dog named Canela at home, and I want to be a veterinarian when I grow up. I dream of taking care of and rescuing street dogs.

**Do you have friends? Can you tell me a story about how they came to be?**

I have a friend named Pablo. We became friends because we both like building things with LEGO. My friend's dad is friends with my dad, and once they came to my house, and we built things with LEGO for hours. Since then, we play together during recess.

**If you were ever told that there was a possibility of becoming neurotypical and leaving Asperger's behind, would you accept leaving Asperger's behind? Why?**

I'm not sure. I like how I think about some things, but sometimes I wish it was easier to make friends. I think I would try it if I could still be myself.

**Are you proud of who you are as a person? What do you consider your purpose in life?**

Yes, I am proud of being good at natural sciences and civic and ethics. I think my purpose is to learn everything I can about dogs and share that knowledge with others.

**Do you have any message for your future readers? And for your future self?**

To others, I would say that it's okay to be different and that everyone has something special to offer. To my future self, I would say to keep pursuing your dreams and never stop learning about the world.

**INTERVIEW #7**

**What is your name?**

My name is José Carlos. I am an architect, and I am 36 years old. I specialize in urban design and landscaping, and I enjoy creating spaces that integrate nature with people's everyday lives.

**Do you consider yourself different from those around you? Why?**

Yes, I consider myself different. My way of seeing and processing the world is distinct. I often focus intensely on details and can spend hours working on a design, perfecting every aspect. While others may easily navigate social situations, I prefer to observe and analyze before interacting. My interests and passions are usually deeper and more specific.

**When did you find out you had Asperger's? How did you find out and what was your reaction to the news?**

I found out I had Asperger's when I was 16 years old. My family and I had noticed that I had difficulties socializing and understanding certain social norms. After several evaluations, a specialist gave us the diagnosis. At first, I felt confused and somewhat scared, but soon I realized that this explained many of my experiences and helped me understand myself better.

**What was/is your life like in school/university?**

In school, I excelled in subjects that interested me, such as mathematics and art, but social interactions were difficult. I preferred spending time in the library or working on personal projects, and I also loved reading architecture books I bought at bookstores. In university, while studying architecture, I found a more welcoming environment. The structure of the studies and the ability to focus on specific projects helped me excel. I made some friends who shared my interests, which made socializing easier.

**Did you ever talk about your disorder with your teachers and/or classmates? If so, how did they react?**

Yes, I spoke with some teachers and classmates about my Asperger's. Most of my teachers were very understanding and tried to adapt their teaching methods to my needs. Over time, I learned to surround myself with people who accepted and supported me.

**Do you prefer solitude or being in the company of others?**

I prefer solitude most of the time because it allows me to focus on my projects and thoughts without interruptions. However, I also enjoy the company of a small group of friends, especially my best friend who, despite being very hyperactive and playful, always makes me smile and gives me a sense of calm when I'm stressed or upset.

**What are your biggest difficulties being Asperger's?**

The biggest difficulties include understanding social cues and handling unexpected changes. Also, at least in the past, I had a lot of trouble expressing what I thought adequately because I would stutter, forget words, or mix up word order due to the nerves of speaking, even though I had rehearsed what I was going to say several times in my mind.

**What are your biggest interests and dreams for the future?**

My biggest interests are sustainable architectural design and landscaping. I dream of creating projects that are not only beautiful but also functional and environmentally friendly. I want to contribute to a world where urban spaces are in harmony with nature and improve people's quality of life. Designing avant-garde buildings and becoming a renowned architect in Monterrey and later in the rest of the country. If possible, I would even try to showcase my works on social media to give them greater visibility in other countries.

**Do you have friends and/or a partner? Can you tell me a story about how they became one?**

Yes, I have a few close friends and a wonderful partner, María. We met in an urban design workshop. At first, we were just colleagues, but soon we discovered that we shared a passion for sustainable architecture. Our friendship grew from there, and over time, it turned into a romantic relationship based on mutual respect and understanding.

**If you were ever told that there is a possibility of becoming neurotypical and leaving Asperger's behind, would you accept leaving Asperger's? Why?**

I don't think I would accept it. Although Asperger's comes with challenges, it has also endowed me with the gift of symmetry and detail perception that my peers can hardly match. I am proud of who I am and know that today I am also a pride to my parents and friends, and that is more than enough for me.

**Are you proud of who you are as a person? What do you consider your purpose in life?**

Yes, I am proud of who I am. My purpose in life is to use my skills and unique perspective to contribute positively to society. I want to help others through architecture and advocate for the acceptance and understanding of people with autism spectrum disorders. I know I still have a long way to go, but for now, I live the life of my dreams, and I know that one day my designs will be an example for future generations.

**Do you have any message to give to your future readers? And to your future self?**

To those who read what we talked about today, I would like to remind you that everyone has a story worth hearing. Never be prejudiced or judge others without truly knowing them because we don't understand the battles each person is fighting at this moment. Be humble and understanding, and I assure you that life will look kindly upon you. As for my future self, I can only say: "You achieved your perfect life."

# Final Chapter: Thank you very much to all my readers!

We have reached the end of this book, and I have nothing left but to deeply thank you for accompanying me on this journey and sharing with you a topic so important and close to my heart. I know that autism can be a difficult subject to tackle and is often surrounded by misunderstandings and prejudices. However, I hope that through these pages we have been able to demystify some of those misconceptions and learn together about the importance of accepting and understanding individuals with Asperger's and autism.

First of all, we have explored and corrected many common misconceptions about autism. One of the most prevalent is the belief that autism is a disease when it is actually a developmental disorder. This misunderstanding can lead to incorrect and often harmful approaches to the treatment and perception of people with autism. It is crucial to understand that autism is not something that needs to be "cured," but a condition that must be understood and accepted.

Another common mistake is the idea that all people with autism are similar, when in reality there is a vast diversity within the autistic spectrum. Each individual with autism is unique, with their own challenges and strengths. Some may need more support in certain areas, while others may be completely independent. This diversity is what makes the autistic spectrum so complex and fascinating.

We have also discussed the negative perception of autism. It is easy to focus on the challenges and difficulties, but it is equally important to recognize and celebrate the many positive things and contributions that people with autism can bring. Throughout this book, I have tried to highlight the extraordinary skills, unique talents, and valuable perspectives that people with autism can offer to our society.

One of the most important messages I want to convey is that people with autism are fully capable of leading normal and fulfilling lives if given the opportunity and proper support. Acceptance and understanding are fundamental. We must strive to create an inclusive environment where all people, regardless of their condition, can thrive and reach their full potential.

Knowledge is power, and learning more about autism and Asperger's is a vital step toward creating a more inclusive and compassionate society. We can expand our understanding through books, conferences, and perhaps most enriching, by getting to know and interacting with people with autism. Each encounter is an opportunity to learn and grow.

People with any degree of autism have extraordinary talents and can achieve incredible things if provided with the right environment. I have seen firsthand how a supportive and understanding environment can transform lives. Imagine a world where every person with autism has access to the opportunities and resources they need to fully develop. The wonders they could achieve are immeasurable.

So today, as we close this book, I encourage you all to accept and understand people with Asperger's, autism, and any other condition within the spectrum. Do not judge or discriminate against anyone because of their condition. Instead, let's celebrate diversity and work together to create a world where everyone has the opportunity to thrive.

Think of it this way: if someone with autism had the same opportunities as anyone else, what wonders could they not achieve? Inclusion and understanding not only benefit people with autism but enrich our entire society.

Thank you very much for accompanying me on this journey. Together, by understanding and accepting autism, we can make the world a better place for everyone. Let us move forward with empathy and the firm conviction that every person, regardless of their differences, has immeasurable value!

## ASPERGER

Everything feels strange, I can't quite grasp,
The world that spins around me.
Understanding's tough, it leaves me in a bind,
I wonder, "Why must it be?"

Details worry me,
Social cues confuse,
I struggle to figure out
How to feel and make friends too.

But I don't lose hope,
I start anew each day,
Facing fears that come to light,
Pain won't keep me at bay.

I am strong to face
The complaints that others bring,
I keep moving forward,
Learning to be myself, I cling.

It's not defeat but a fight,
That neither stops nor breaks my will,
It makes me stronger inside,
And with courage, I face Asperger still.


## AUTISM

Being autistic isn't a disease,
It's a unique way to see the world with ease.
There are countless ways to be on the spectrum,
Each comes with its own set of challenges and them.

Sometimes language can be a trial,
Even if the heart is warm and worthwhile.
Others may follow many strict rules,
Even if adapting seems like a daunting duel.

There's Asperger's and emotional regulation,
Needing patience and understanding's dedication.
Or ASD with its challenges to perceive,
Causing clashes in how we all receive.

But an autistic person's like you and me,
Deserving love and empathy.
Don't judge what you don't understand,
For an autistic person's human, just like all in the land.


## ATTENTION DEFICIT HYPERACTIVITY DISORDER

At times, the mind feels lost in thought,
And focus seems like something hard-fought.
While the urge for action never ceases,
And restlessness brings no easy pieces.

It's ADHD, a constant sway,
That keeps on impacting day by day.
A path of highs and lows we tread,
Navigating challenges with each step ahead.

Ideas burst forth, nonstop and free,
Getting into trouble often seems to be.
Restlessness, chaos, and the pain it brings,
Living through tears with the struggles it sings.

Yet despite every challenge and trial,
View life from a different angle with a smile.
Show the strength you hold within,
And success is still within reach to win.


## RETT SYNDROME

I felt trapped with no way out,
Wondering if the light was just a doubt.
With Rett, my life took a drastic turn,
As my mind and spirit began to churn.

I faced the challenges that came my way,
To break free from the block that led me astray.

Searching for a solution, I would rise,
Yet my despair often clouded my skies.

It felt like the world was crashing down,
But my family's love was my solid ground.
Now that I've faced the trials surrounding me,
I find that nothing is too complex to see.

Rett Syndrome, though it's tough to bear,
Only makes me stronger with each trial I dare.


## OPPOSITIONAL DEFIANT DISORDER

Oppositional defiant disorder
Affects many of us,
When it comes to relating
And giving without fuss.

Our anger has no reason,
We respond with hostility,
With shouting and outbursts
In a quest for control.

We feel oppressed
And sometimes frustrated,
Though everything angers us
And we provoke tantrums.

It's a difficult condition,
That prevents us from understanding,
That with love and respect
We can receive a helping hand.

Let's close the door on our anger,
And open our hearts,
To find balance
And a profound sense of well-being.

## OBSESSIVE-COMPULSIVE DISORDER

Occasionally I yield to the disorder
My busy mind and soul affected
Obsessions here, compulsions there
The struggle turns, a challenge to the end.

The voice whispers, "Do all you can"
Better do it again to release the power
Obligations always in the way
Even the slightest neglect can increase the fear.

Trapped in the wheel, the fight always changing
Attempts to overcome, but my hope is fading
Raining every day with my obsessions and compulsions,
And yet, I have a reason to keep going.

I hope the day comes when my struggle for freedom becomes reality.


## FRAGILE X SYNDROME

To a child with Fragile X Syndrome
Sad is the life, your effort always ignored,
Tears stream down your lonely, sorrowful face,
Your understanding slow, your body unsteady,
Lacking the strength to face your challenges.

Yet, your fate is not unchangeable,
Love and support you will find if you seek,
Life may be tough, but you are a survivor,
A true hero, an indomitable force.

You will show your skills, give your best,
Ignore the harsh and cruel comments,
You will challenge your mind and body,
And from your situation, make a flower.

Your struggles may seem impossible to overcome
And your limits may feel near,
But your courage will conquer obstacles,
And you will make your dreams come true.

Oh, Fragile X Syndrome
A difficult challenge to face,
Your destiny is not unchangeable,
The possibilities are indeed infinite.

## SENSORY INTEGRATION DISORDER

Separated from reality,
something eludes me.
Five senses push me to the edge,
making my life a deep abyss.

With noise, light, and strong touches,
the stimuli overwhelm me.
I fall halfway through the path,
feeling unsettled and alone.

My world, a desolate ruin,
no response I expect.
Submerged in the vastness,
my soul finds no peace.

Uncertainty weighs me down,
everything is an enigma.
And every day reminds me
of the tragedy of my sensory integration disorder.

# Final Acknowledgments

First and foremost, I want to express my deepest gratitude to my family. Despite the ups and downs we have faced in the past, they have always been by my side, supporting me every step of the way. They have sacrificed time, effort, and money to provide me with a career, an education, and, above all, values that remain a fundamental part of my life to this day. Their love and dedication have been the foundation upon which I have built my achievements, and without them, none of this would have been possible. Thank you for being my rock and my constant inspiration. Every sacrifice, every word of encouragement, and every gesture of love have shaped me into the person I am today. They have been my refuge in times of storm and my guide in moments of uncertainty. There are not enough words to express my gratitude for everything they have done for me.

I also want to thank my teachers Alicia Castillo and Ahelí de Alba. They not only motivated me to work hard to get ahead in life but also inspired me to write this book. Their passion for teaching and their faith in my abilities have guided me in moments of doubt and pushed me to reach new goals. Alicia and Ahelí, thank you for your dedication, for believing in me, and for igniting the spark of writing in me. This book is as much yours as it is mine, and I am eternally grateful for your influence in my life. Your teachings have transcended the classroom and have become life lessons that I carry with me every day. Your words of encouragement have been a beacon of light in the darkest moments, and your commitment to my success has been a constant source of inspiration.

Finally, I want to express my sincere gratitude to my friends. They have played a very important role in my life, and although we have faced various problems at times, they have always advised, inspired, supported, and, most importantly, tolerated me. The friendship we share has been a pillar of strength and joy, and I deeply value every moment shared with you. I am very grateful to have you in my life and am sure that together we will achieve great things in the future. Your presence has enriched my life in ways that words cannot fully express. Every shared laugh, every shoulder to lean on, and every heartfelt piece of advice have been invaluable treasures that I deeply cherish. You have shown me the true meaning of friendship and have been my chosen family in the most crucial moments of my life.

Additionally, I would like to extend my gratitude to all the people who have been a part of my journey, directly or indirectly. To those who offered a kind word, to the mentors who provided wisdom and guidance, and to the companions who shared their own stories and experiences. Every interaction, every small act of kindness, has left an indelible mark on my heart and contributed to my personal and professional growth. The community surrounding me has been a fabric of support and strength, and I am incredibly grateful for every thread that composes this tapestry of my life.

Thank you all, my family, my teachers, my friends, and every person who has crossed my path. Your love, support, and guidance have been essential in my journey, and I dedicate this book to you with all my heart. This achievement is not just mine, but belongs to all those who have believed in me and supported me along the way. Thank you, from the bottom of my heart! May this book be a testament to the strength of community, the importance of mutual support, and the beauty of human connections.